3

Reflexology

Thorsons First Directions

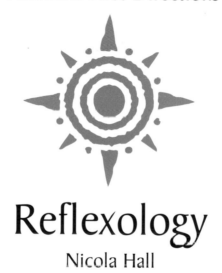

Reflexology

Nicola Hall

Thorsons
An imprint of HarperCollins*Publishers*
77–85 Fulham Palace Road
Hammersmith, London W6 8JB

The Thorsons website address is:
www.thorsons.com

Published by Thorsons in 2001
Text derived from *Principles of Reflexology*, published by Thorsons, 1996
10 9 8 7 6 5 4 3 2 1

Text copyright© Nicola M. Hall 2001
Copyright© HarperCollins*Publishers* Ltd 2001

Editor: Jo Kyle
Design: Wheelhouse Creative
Production: Melanie Vandevelde
Photography: PhotoDisc Europe

Nicola M. Hall asserts the moral right to be identified as author of this work

A catalogue record for this book is available from the British Library

ISBN 0 00 713028 7

Printed and bound in Hong Kong

Contents

Reflexology

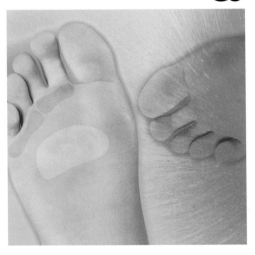

is the practice of applying pressure to reflex
stimulate the body's own healing system

points in the feet and hands to

What is Reflexology?

Today reflexology refers to a method of treatment whereby reflex points in the feet are massaged in a particular way to bring about an effect in areas of the body quite distant from the feet. There are also similar reflex points to be found in the hands, which may also be used for treatment, but where possible it is preferable to work on the foot reflexes since the response is better. Reflexology is derived from a treatment that was originally known as 'zone therapy', a term that is sometimes still used.

History of the method

The origins of reflexology date back at least 5000 years to when the Chinese were known to have practised a form of pressure therapy with

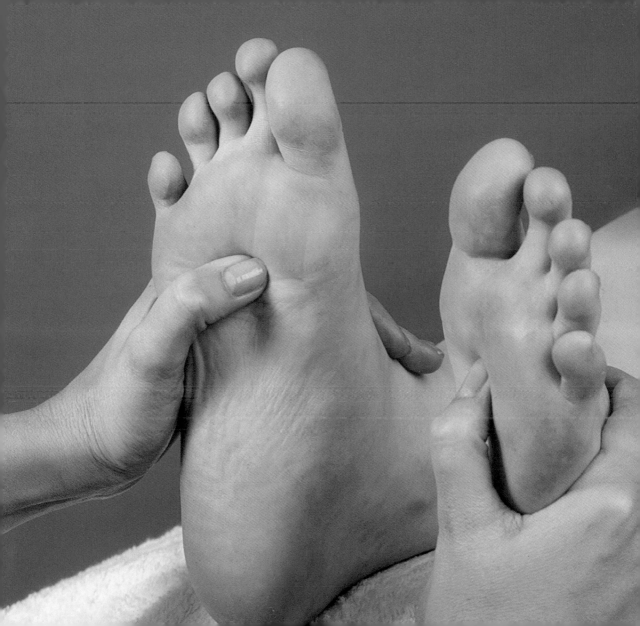

a basis similar to that of acupuncture. The ancient Egyptians were also known to be using similar methods in about 3000 BC. We see this illustrated in tomb drawings where the feet were being held and massaged in a particular way.

One of the earliest books to be written on the subject of zone therapy was published in 1582 by two eminent European physicians called Dr Adamus and Dr A'tatis. Another book on the same subject was also published shortly after this in Leipzig by a Dr Bell and it is known that at this time many people in the middle European countries from the poor to the wealthy, including royalty, all used a form of pressure therapy. In more recent times there has been evidence that some of the Red Indian tribes and primitive tribes of Africa have been using a form of reflexology.

The first real advancement of zone therapy can, however, be attributed to an American physician and surgeon from Connecticut called Dr William H. Fitzgerald.

The Findings of Dr Fitzgerald

In 1913, Dr Fitzgerald commenced his research into the method of healing which he termed zone therapy. At the time he was head of the Nose and Throat department of the St Francis Hospital in Hartford and was well respected as a medical surgeon and physician.

Dr Fitzgerald had initially been intrigued by the fact that at times he was able to carry out an operation on the nose and throat without the patient experiencing much pain, while at other times a similar operation on a different patient caused considerable pain. He found that in the cases where little pain was felt, the patient had been applying pressure on certain parts of the hand or that during the examination prior to the operation, he himself had applied pressure to certain areas and these pressures had inhibited pain in other areas. With time, Fitzgerald traced these locations and described how the body could be divided into ten longitudinal zones – five on each side of a median line through the body. Each zone related to one of the five digits on each side of the body, with zone one extending from the big toe up the entire body to the brain and down the arm to the thumb, zone two extending from the second toe up to the brain and down to the second finger, zone three extending from the third toe up to the brain and down to the third finger, zone four extending from the fourth toe up to the brain and down to the fourth finger and zone five, the outer zone, extending from the fifth toe up to the brain and down to the fifth or little finger. All of these zones extended right through the body from front to back and rather than being single lines, they were sections through the body of equal width. The zones did not cross in the head, as with nerves, so that the right side of the head and brain related to corresponding zones on the right side of the body and the left side of the head and brain related to corresponding zones on the left side of the body. By applying pressure to an area or areas in a certain zone, it was possible to inhibit pain in other areas within the same zone.

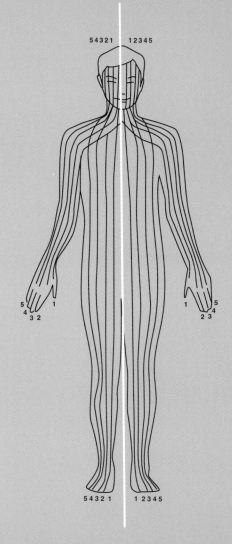

The zones of the body

Other pioneers of the method

The work of Dr Fitzgerald was first publicised by Dr Edwin F. Bowers who was a medical critic and writer from New York. The medical world did not respond very favourably to this new method but more support was found from practitioners of natural medicine such as chiropractors, osteopaths and naturopaths. However, there was some interest from fellow doctors, some of whom researched the subject further and made valuable contributions to the development of the method. These persons included Dr George Starr White, Dr Joe Riley and his wife Elizabeth Riley. Dr Riley wrote many books on the subject and also introduced the use of 'hook work'. 'Hook work' was so called because it involved the fingers of the practitioner being hooked over some part of the body of the patient in order to manipulate that area.

Another great pioneer in the field was an American lady called Eunice D. Ingham. Having trained with Dr Riley, Eunice Ingham developed the 'Ingham Compression Method of Reflexology'. She wrote two books called *Stories the Feet Can Tell* and *Stories the Feet Have Told*, which became standard textbooks for reflexology students. Eunice Ingham had trained as a remedial therapist so had a para-medical background and she devoted herself in her later years to reflexology and the promotion of the method. In addition to a highly successful

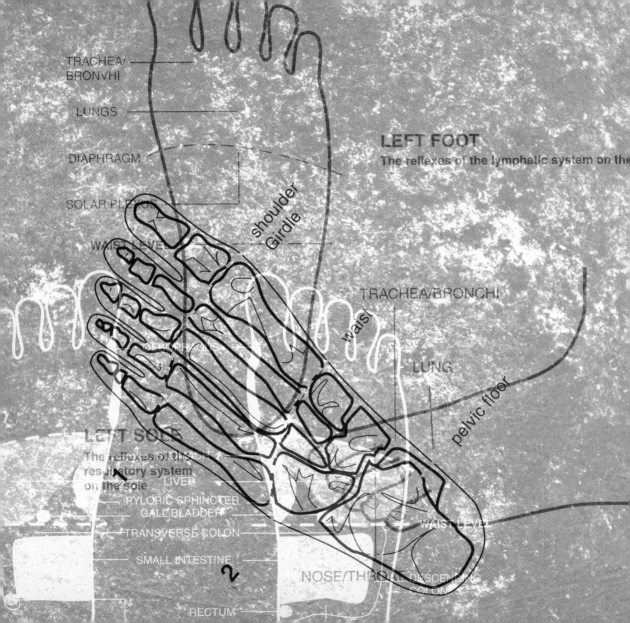

TRACHEA/
BRONVHI

LUNGS

DIAPHRAGM

SOLAR PLEXUS

WAIST LEVEL

shoulder
Girdle

LEFT FOOT

The reflexes of the lymphatic system on the

TRACHEA/BRONCHI

waist

LUNG

pelvic floor

LEFT SOLE

The reflexes of the
respiratory system
on the sole

STOMACH

LIVER

PYLORIC SPHINCTER

GALL BLADDER

TRANSVERSE COLON

SMALL INTESTINE

WAIST LEVEL

2

NOSE/THROAT DESCENDING
COLON

RECTUM

practice, she toured America extensively, lecturing, treating and teaching new practitioners.

The main pioneer of the work in Great Britain was Mrs Doreen E. Bayly who in her younger years had trained as a nurse. Mrs Bayly met Eunice Ingham while on a visit to her sister in America. She was greatly impressed by her work and studied with Eunice Ingham before returning to England in the early 1960s. After much perseverance, Mrs Bayly created more interest in reflexology in Britain and on the Continent and built up a busy practice as well as starting a training school for reflexology. She died in 1979 at a time when reflexology was beginning to gain more acclaim. Her teachings are still continued through the Bayly School of Reflexology.

Reflexology today

Reflexology has developed from the initial practice of zone therapy and in present times most practitioners of the method will concentrate on treating by massage to the reflex areas in the feet. The reflexes in the hands may also be used in some instances, but generally the reflexes in the feet are considered more responsive.

Reflexology is a method which people often feel they can apply to themselves with just a little knowledge of the subject, but the best results will be obtained when a trained practitioner gives treatment.

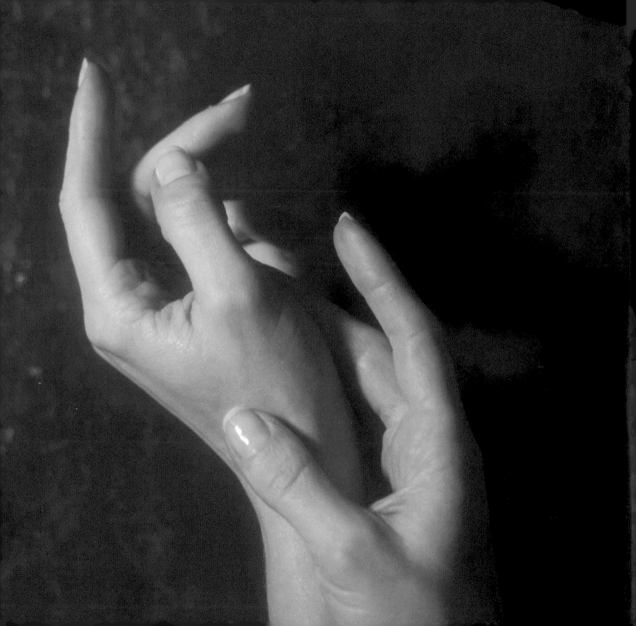

How the Treatment Works

To many people, the idea of massaging the feet to improve their health seems too far-fetched to be taken seriously, but it is possible through reflexology treatment to help many disorders. As previously mentioned, in the feet and the hands there are reflex areas relating to all the parts of the body, so the whole body may be treated through the feet. Every part of the foot corresponds to a part of the body, with reflex areas being found on the soles of the feet and also on the top and sides of the feet. The hands, likewise, contain reflex areas on the palms and the backs of the hands.

The zone systems

The arrangement of the reflex points in the feet is such that they provide a logical map of the body; this organization of points is based on the zone system which exists in the body as described by Dr Fitzgerald. The ten longitudinal zones, as explained in the previous chapter, extend throughout the body with five zones on either side of a median or central line. These zones are not lines, such as the acupuncture meridian lines, but are sections through the body of equal width and extending from front to back. Whichever zone or zones of the body an organ exists in, there will be a corresponding reflex area in the same zone or zones of the feet. Remembering that these zones do not cross in the brain, as does the nervous system, the right side of the body is represented in the right foot and the left side of the body is represented in the left foot.

In addition to the ten longitudinal zones originally described, it has also been found that three transverse zones exist in the body, which can also be described in the feet. These transverse zones can be seen in the body by drawing three imaginary lines as follows:

1. a line drawn across the upper shoulder girdle.
2. a line drawn across at waist level at the lower level of the ribs.
3. a line drawn across the level of the pelvic floor.

The area above line one relates to the structures of the head and neck. The area between lines one and two relates to the structures of the thorax and upper abdomen. The area between lines two and three relates to the structures of the abdomen and pelvis. These areas can be transposed onto the feet and relate to the skeletal structure of the feet.

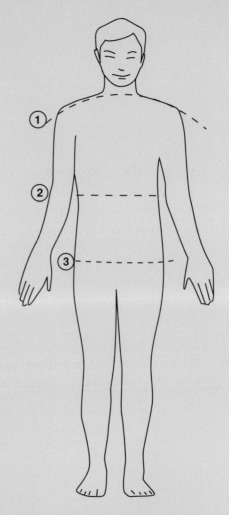

The transverse zones of the body

The structure of the foot

Each foot is made up of 26 bones; associated with the bones are 19 muscles and 107 ligaments. Each foot has 14 phalanges, which are the bones of the toes, with each toe being made up of three bones, except for the big toe which has just two bones. Leading back from the toes towards the heel are five bones called metatarsals, with one relating to each toe. The remaining bones of the feet are called the tarsal bones with three cuneiform bones, a cuboid bone, a navicular bone, a talus bone and a calcaneum bone (the heelbone).

From this bony structure of the foot, it is now possible to see how the transverse zones of the body relate to the bones of the feet.

Line 1 is at the base of the phalanges so that the reflexes of the head and neck are found in the toe areas.

Line 2 is at the base of the metatarsal bones so the reflexes of the thorax and upper abdomen are found in the area over the metatarsal bones.

Line 3 is across the tarsal bones up to and including the ankle bones (inner and outer malleoli) so the reflexes to the abdomen and pelvis are found over the tarsal bones and around the ankle bones.

With the presence of both longitudinal and transverse zones in the body and the fact that these zones can be transposed onto the feet,

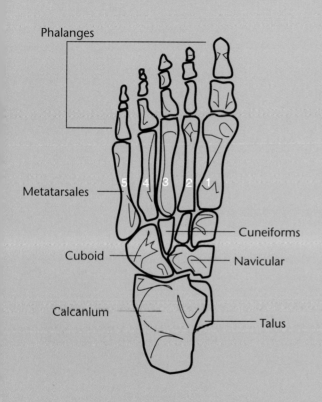

Phalanges

Metatarsales

Cuboid

Calcanium

Cuneiforms

Navicular

Talus

5 4 3 2 1

The bones of the foot

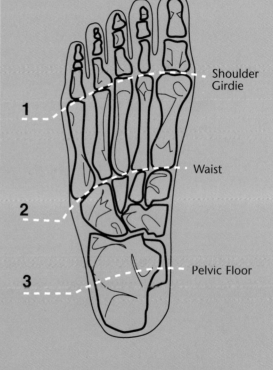

Shoulder
Girdie

Waist

Pelvic Floor

1

2

3

**The transverse zones
of the foot**

there exists in the feet a 'grid-like' system which aids in the determination of the positions of the various reflex areas. There are a few slight exceptions to this pattern and these will be mentioned at a later stage, but for the majority of areas the zone pattern holds true.

How does it work?

The exact reactions that take place when an area of the foot is massaged, resulting in an effect on a part of the body to which the area of the foot corresponds, are not fully understood. Various theories have been put forward to explain the workings of reflexology and some of the more common theories will now be discussed.

In very simple terms it is accepted that reflexology can have an effect on the blood circulation and the nervous system. A healthy circulation is vital for healthy functioning of all the body parts, with the blood transporting the necessary nutrients to the tissues and then carrying away from the tissues the waste products of metabolism. Reflexology can improve the circulation to all areas and thus help this important transport system in the body to work to its fullest potential, in turn assisting the various body systems to function better.

With the nervous system, it is accepted that approximately 70 per cent of all disorders are due to 'nerve tension' in the different areas of

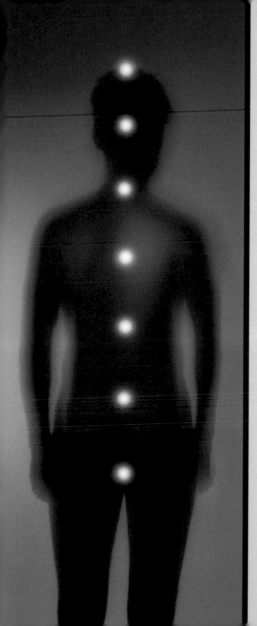

the body and reflexology can be most
effective in helping to reduce this tension,
thus enabling the different areas to become
more 'relaxed' and therefore function more
efficiently. With many simple disorders the
body is able to right itself without
medication since it has a tremendous power
to heal itself. Reflexology is able to help
stimulate the healing forces present in the
body and thus aid the body in its self-
treatment.

Within the longitudinal zones described it
is known that there is a flow of energy linking
the organs within the same zone. The exact
type of energy involved is not yet
understood, though work is being done in
this field in relation to the various forms of
ancient Chinese medicine which work on
energy systems. By the means of Kirlian
photography, which is able to show the
energy fields surrounding objects, it has
been shown that the energy field or corona

present around the reflex areas in the feet will be diminished when there is an imbalance in the body area corresponding to the reflex area. This corona will become improved or corrected, and therefore more defined, after reflexology treatment has been given, showing that the treatment has successfully balanced the energy field.

The pain-reducing effect of reflexology may possibly be explained by the ability of massage of the reflex areas to cause the release of substances, known as endorphins, from the brain. Endorphins act as the body's natural pain-relieving agents.

In certain reflex areas in the feet, crystal-like deposits may be felt by the practitioner. These crystals are presumed to be made up of calcium deposits which settle beneath the skin surface at the nerve endings in the feet. These crystals feel to the practitioner like pieces of grit or gravel beneath the skin surface and by massaging these 'gritty' areas the crystals can be broken down and then be more easily removed by the blood circulation. Some authorities have stated that these crystals will always be felt in the feet when there is imbalance in the corresponding body area and that reflexology is all about dispersing the crystals. Although these crystals are often felt, it is not necessarily the case and reflex areas in the feet may indicate imbalances in the body without 'gritty' areas being present.

Whatever the correct scientific explanation for reflexology, and it may well be many years before the treatment can be fully explained, the fact that the method does work can be seen by the number of people who have received treatment and benefited from it – surely good enough evidence for many to justify trying it.

Balancing effect

The work of reflexology is to balance up all the systems of the body and harmonize the entire organism. The term 'out of balance' is used to imply that a particular area is not functioning efficiently either due to poor circulation to that area or tension in that area. Because the overall effect of the treatment is to balance, an overactive area will be calmed and an underactive area will be stimulated until the balance in the body is restored. The body is so easily thrown 'out of balance' by stress, diet or negative thoughts, and the resulting imbalances, even if only slight, will prevent 100 per cent efficiency of all the body functions. The imbalances are due to blockages in the flow of energy throughout the body. When working on the reflex areas in the feet, imbalances can be detected and by treating these areas the body can be brought back into balance leading to better health.

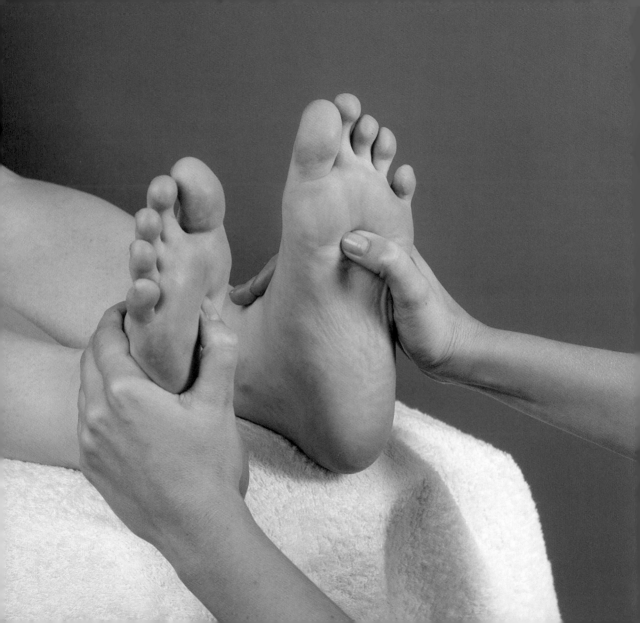

How the Treatment is Given

The first visit to somewhere new is frequently a slightly anxious experience for many people and especially when it also involves treatment of illness. Reflexology treatment is certainly not an unpleasant experience so should not provoke any additional anxieties! Often people are worried that the treatment is going to be very painful but again this should not be the case if the method is applied correctly by a reputable practitioner.

Medical history

On the first visit to a practitioner, a detailed medical history of the new patient will be taken. This is helpful to the practitioner not only in assisting with the treatment procedure but also in making sure that no symptoms exist which would prevent treatment from being administered. Any serious illnesses or operations will be enquired about and a patient should not feel embarrassed to mention any of these, however many, since they are all relevant to the complete health of that person.

Treatment position

Once a medical history has been recorded, the patient will be asked to sit, ideally in a reclining chair, which will be tipped back after the removal of the patient's shoes and socks. This is the best position for a patient to be in, with the back comfortably supported and with the lower leg from knee to ankle also supported so that the feet can be rested in a relaxed and comfortable position. If the knee is not bent and the leg is straight, the foot tends to be held more tensely, which hampers the treatment. When the patient is comfortably positioned, the treatment session will begin.

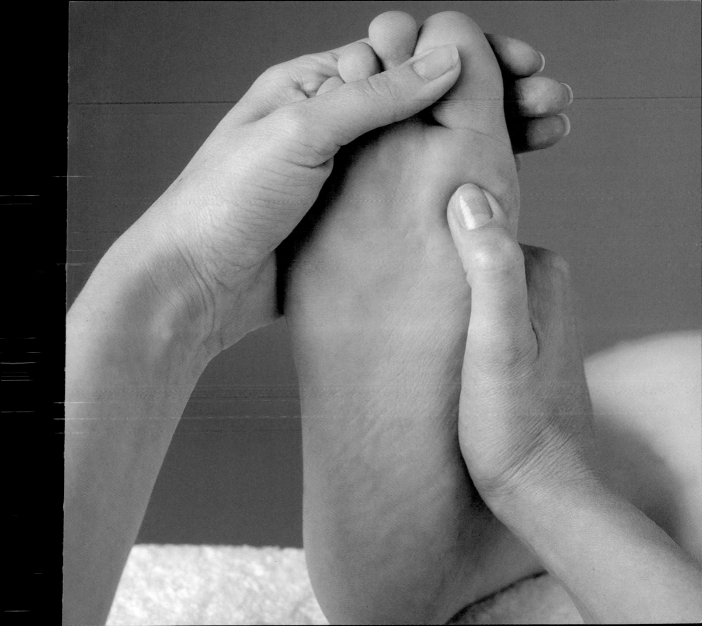

Both hands may be used and it is quite common for the practitioner to switch from using the right thumb to using the left thumb as it is easier to reach certain areas on each foot with one or other hand. It is important that the pressure applied is not painful to the patient as this would immediately make him/her tense. The pressure will be firm but always bearable.

Usually a pattern of treatment will be followed, commencing with massage of the right foot with the reflexes to be found in the region of the big toe. The whole foot will then be systematically treated, working down from the toes across the areas on the sole of the foot down to the heel. The areas on the sides and top of the foot will then be treated before carrying out the same procedure on the left foot.

At the end of a complete treatment both feet will be given some gentle manipulation and the movements generally applied include rotation of the toes, rotation of the ankles, a kneading action with the fist on the sole of the foot and a 'wringing' action with the hands cupped around the sides of the feet, rotating away from each other. The treatment session will finish with a relaxing breathing exercise where the thumbs are placed over the reflexes to the solar plexus; as the patient breathes in pressure is applied to the reflexes and the feet pushed up gently towards the body and as the patient breathes out the pressure is released and the feet pulled gently away from the body.

massage

relaxing

breathing

pressure

kneading

rotation

What the treatment feels like

In different parts of the feet, different reactions are felt. Some areas, when massaged, may feel as if something very sharp, like a piece of glass or a thorn, is being pressed into the foot. In other areas the massage may produce a feeling of slight discomfort, and in areas where definite crystals are present beneath the skin surface, the patient may be aware of these 'gritty' areas being worked on and slowly broken down by the practitioner.

If there is much tension present in the body it is not surprising to find very many tender areas in the feet, but those areas that are most tender will indicate which parts of the body are most out of balance.

Reactions from the treatment

Directly after a treatment session has finished the feet should feel warm and the patient should feel very relaxed. It is best that the patient does not go dashing about directly after treatment to allow the relaxed state to continue and thus allow the healing processes in the body to take place more readily.

There will be no unpleasant side effects from reflexology. It is possible, however, for some form of healing crisis to occur as the body attempts to heal itself and rid itself of toxic substances. Because of the possibility of a reaction to treatment occurring, the first treatment session will always be given quite gently to see how the person reacts. The different forms of healing crisis will mainly affect the eliminating systems of the body, which may show increased activity. These include the kidneys, the bowels, the skin and the lungs. Reactions should be considered as positive factors, will be short-term and are indications that the body is attempting to become more balanced.

Number of treatments required

For all conditions a course of treatment is required and even if just one session appears to have corrected the problem it is more sensible to have a short course of treatment to help balance up totally the body systems and to help prevent a recurrence of the disorder. For most conditions, a course of six to eight treatments is advisable and treatment sessions will usually take place at weekly intervals. Treatment may sometimes be given twice a week, particularly in conditions such as back problems, where the injury has just occurred and where considerable pain is being experienced. To treat more frequently than once or, on occasions twice, a week is not recommended since there is always the possibility of over-working an area and causing too strong a reaction in the body. It must be remembered that the body needs time to try to balance up the systems and for repair work to be done.

Treatment time

The length of time for each treatment session varies but, since with every treatment all the reflex areas in both feet must be treated to treat the whole body, this will take about three-quarters of an hour. In certain cases, for example if the patient has extremely sensitive or very tense feet, it is necessary to work more slowly, and the treatment session may last up to one hour, but to work for much longer than one hour is excessive.

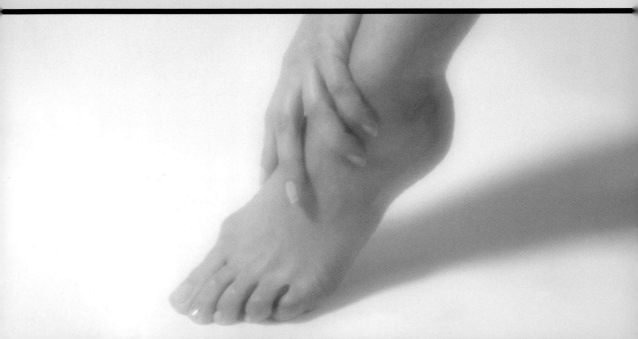

The Reflex Areas

The way that the body can be divided into ten longitudinal and three transverse zone areas has already been described, as well as how these zones help to determine the position of the various reflex areas in the feet. The illustration overleaf shows the anatomical arrangement of the different parts of the body and the longitudinal zones in which these different parts are situated. The arrangement of the reflex areas in the feet will now be looked at more closely by considering the different systems of the body as follows:

1. The head areas
2. The musculo-skeletal system
3. The endocrine system
4. The respiratory system
5. The heart and circulatory system
6. The lymphatic system
7. The digestive system
8. The urinary system
9. The skin

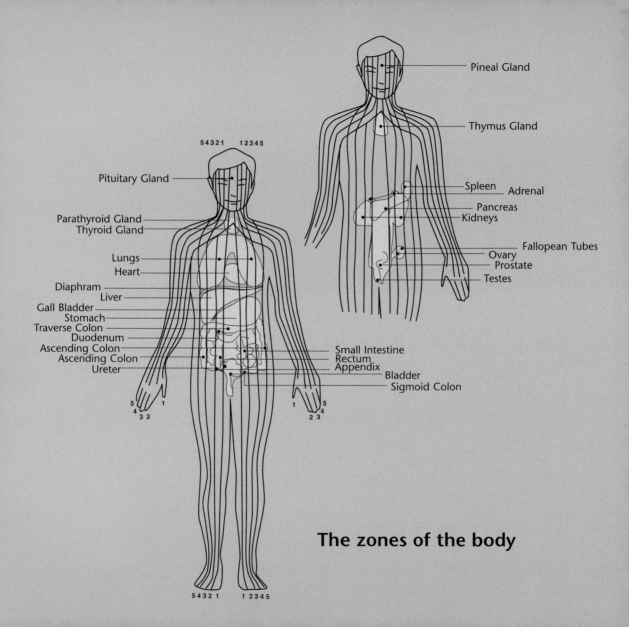

54321 12345

Pineal Gland

Thymus Gland

Pituitary Gland

Spleen — Adrenal
Pancreas
Kidneys

Parathyroid Gland
Thyroid Gland

Fallopean Tubes
Ovary
Prostate
Testes

Lungs
Heart
Diaphram
Liver
Gall Bladder
Stomach
Traverse Colon
Duodenum
Ascending Colon
Ascending Colon
Ureter

Small Intestine
Rectum
Appendix
Bladder
Sigmoid Colon

5   1
4
3 2

1   5
4
2 3

The zones of the body

54321 12345

I. The head areas

All the reflexes to the areas of the head are found in the regions of the toes, with the big toes also corresponding to all of the head and each big toe representing five zones.

The brain is part of the central nervous system of the body and is a most complex computer controlling a vast number of bodily functions. The brain is composed of a right and left hemisphere, with the right lobe controlling the left side of the body and the left lobe controlling the right side of the body. However, with reflexology the zone areas do not cross in the brain so that the right side of the brain is represented on the right foot and the left side of the brain is represented on the left foot.

   The reflex areas to the brain are found in the pads of the big toes, with the pituitary gland reflex approximately in the centre of the pad of the big toe and the top of the brain and top of the head reflex areas found at the top of the big toe just behind the nail. The reflex to the side of the brain and side of the head is found down the side of the big toe on the side nearest the second toe. The reflex to the face is found on the top surface of the big toe.

The sinuses are hollow air-filled spaces in the cheekbones and behind the eyebrows and are linked with the nose. They are involved in giving resonance to the voice and also act as a protection to the eyes and the brain.

The reflexes to the sinuses are found in all four small toes on both feet not only all the way up the backs of these toes but sometimes also being more pronounced up the sides of the toes. Since the sinuses are found in zones two to five in the body, the reflexes are found in zones two to five in the feet.

The eyes are the organs of vision. The reflex to the eyes is found at the base of the second and third toes just below where these toes join the sole of the foot. The eyes in the body are situated in zones two and three so the reflexes in the feet are found in zones two and three, with the right eye represented in the right foot and the left eye represented in the left foot.

The ears are the organs of hearing. The reflex to the ears is similarly placed to that of the reflex to the eyes but beneath the fourth and fifth toes. The reflexes are thus in zones four and five, with the right ear reflex represented in the right foot and the left ear reflex represented in the left foot.

The Eustachian tube connects the middle ear to the back of the throat and helps keep the air in the middle ear at atmospheric pressure.

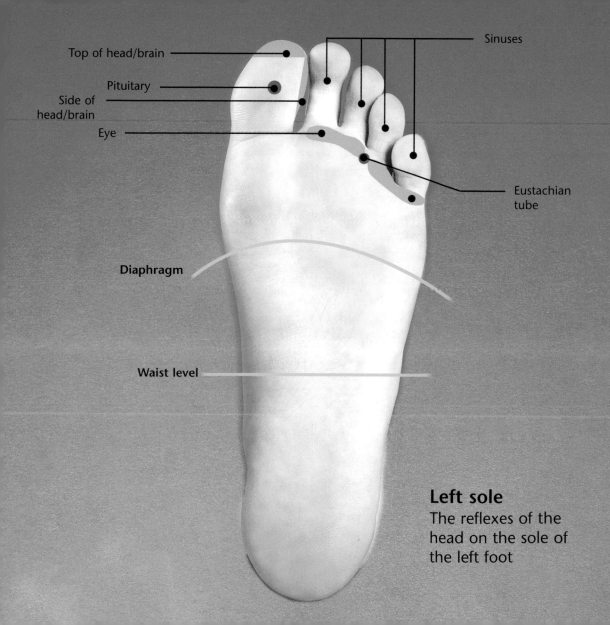

Top of head/brain

Pituitary

Side of
head/brain

Eye

Sinuses

Eustachian
tube

Diaphragm

Waist level

Left sole
The reflexes of the
head on the sole of
the left foot

The reflex to the Eustachian tube is found on the sole of the foot just below the web between the third and fourth toes. It can also be found in a similar position on the top of the foot below the web between the third and fourth toes. The reflex is present on right and left feet.

2. The musculo-skeletal system

This system covers the joints of the body and their associated muscles and includes the spine, the neck, the shoulder girdles, the elbows, the wrists, the pelvic girdles, the hips, the knees and the ankles.

The spine consists of a number of bony segments called vertebrae which can be divided into groups counting downwards, with seven cervical, twelve thoracic, five lumbar, five sacral and four coccygeal vertebrae. In the adult, the sacral and coccygeal vertebrae are fused to form two immobile bones called the sacrum and the coccyx (the tailbone). The bony skeleton of the spine surrounds the spinal cord which is an extension of the brain and the nerves which originate from the spinal cord are named according to the region of the spine from which they emerge. These nerves affect the areas of the body on a level with the region of the spine from which they emerge. Thus the cervical nerves affect the neck and arms, the thoracic nerves affect the chest,

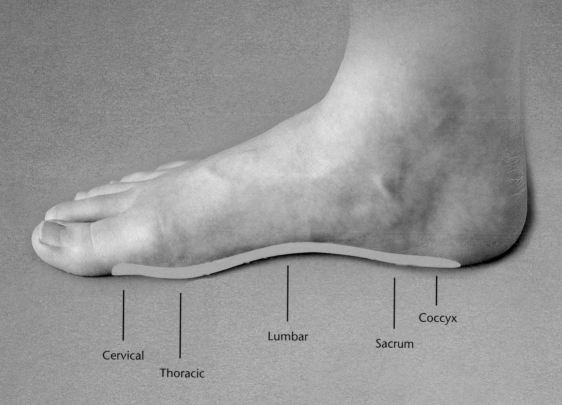

Right Foot
The reflexes of the
spine on the side of
the right foot

Cervical

Thoracic

Lumbar

Sacrum

Coccyx

the lumbar nerves affect the lower extremities such as the legs and feet, the sacral nerves affect the organs of the pelvis and the buttocks and the coccygeal nerves affect the rectum and anus.

The reflex to the spine is found down the inner side of both feet since the spine is situated centrally in the body. The different regions of the spine will be represented accordingly, with the cervical area starting at the top of the side of the big toe and ending level with the base of the big toe. The reflex to the neck is found all around the base of the big toe. The thoracic region of the spine will be represented along the side of the first metatarsal bone, with the lumbar region from the waistline of the foot down to approximately level with the inner ankle bone, and the remaining area along the inner side of the foot representing the region of the sacrum and coccyx.

The upper limbs have three main joints: the shoulders, the elbows and the wrists, as well as the joints of the fingers.

The reflex to the shoulder is found around the base of the fifth (little) toe on the sole of the foot, the outer side of the foot and the top of the foot. The reflex area relating to the shoulder girdle will be found across the sole of the foot and the top of the foot in all five zones. The reflex area will cover the upper half of the metatarsal bones. The reflex to the sternum (breastbone) is found on the top of the foot at the top end of the first metatarsal bone in zone one.

The reflex to the upper arm can be found on the outer side of the foot, slightly on top of the foot leading down from the shoulder reflex to the base of the fifth metatarsal bone (the slight bony projection at waist level on the outer side of the foot), and the elbow reflex will be found at the base of the fifth metatarsal bone.

The pelvis is a large basin-shaped cavity formed by the sacrum and coccyx behind and by the innominate bones (the large bones which are the hip bones) at the front and sides. Within the pelvis are contained the bladder, rectum and reproductive organs which it protects. The reflexes to the pelvic areas are found over the tarsal bones of the feet and the ankle bones.

The reflex to the hip is found below the outer ankle bone and along the outer side of the foot mainly in a half-moon shaped area from half way between the base of the fifth metatarsal bone and the heel to the back of the heel. The hip reflex also relates to the reflex area for the upper leg.

The reflex to the knee is also found on the outer side of the foot in a half-moon shaped area from the base of the fifth metatarsal bone to where the hip reflex starts. The knee reflex also relates to the reflex area for the lower leg.

The reflex to the sacro-iliac joint (where the sacrum of the spine joins with the ilium of the pelvis) is found slightly on top of the foot in

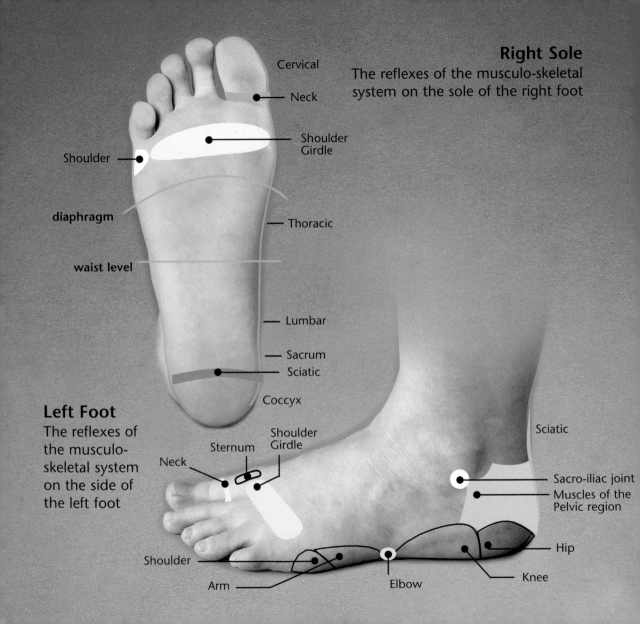

Right Sole
The reflexes of the musculo-skeletal system on the sole of the right foot

Cervical

Neck

Shoulder Girdle

Shoulder

diaphragm

Thoracic

waist level

Lumbar

Sacrum

Sciatic

Coccyx

Left Foot
The reflexes of the musculo-skeletal system on the side of the left foot

Neck

Sternum

Shoulder Girdle

Sciatic

Sacro-iliac joint

Muscles of the Pelvic region

Shoulder

Arm

Elbow

Knee

Hip

a small dip which is often found just in front of the outer ankle bone.

When referring to the reflex areas to the joints, the muscles associated with these joints may also be reached by massaging the corresponding joint areas. Hence, the muscles of the buttock and around the top of the leg will be associated with the reflex areas to the sacro-iliac joints and hips.

The sciatic nerve is the largest nerve in the body and arises from the lower spine and then passes across the buttock, down the back of the leg and divides behind the knee into two main branches supplying the lower leg.

The reflex to the sciatic nerve is found approximately one-third of the way down the slightly hardened base of the heel on the sole of the foot and is present in all five zones. A further reflex area may also be found extending from the edges of this area across the side of the foot and up the back of the leg on either side of the Achilles tendon for a distance of a few inches.

3. The endocrine system

The endocrine system is the hormonal system of the body and plays a very important role in regulating body functions. Endocrine glands are sometimes called ductless glands since their secretions do not pass down ducts to where they are to act but instead are carried in the bloodstream around the body to the various parts of the body which are to be affected. The endocrine glands include the pituitary, the thyroid, the parathyroids, the adrenals, the pancreas and the reproductive glands.

The pituitary is often referred to as the master gland of the body since it helps control the action of many of the other glands in the body. The hormones produced by the pituitary help control growth and affect the secretions of the thyroid, adrenals and reproductive glands, as well as having many other functions.

The reflex to the pituitary gland is found in the centre of the pad of the big toe, though it may vary slightly in position, being somewhat higher or lower or more to one side. A reflex to the pituitary will be found in both big toes.

The thyroid is a two-lobed gland situated in the neck. The main role

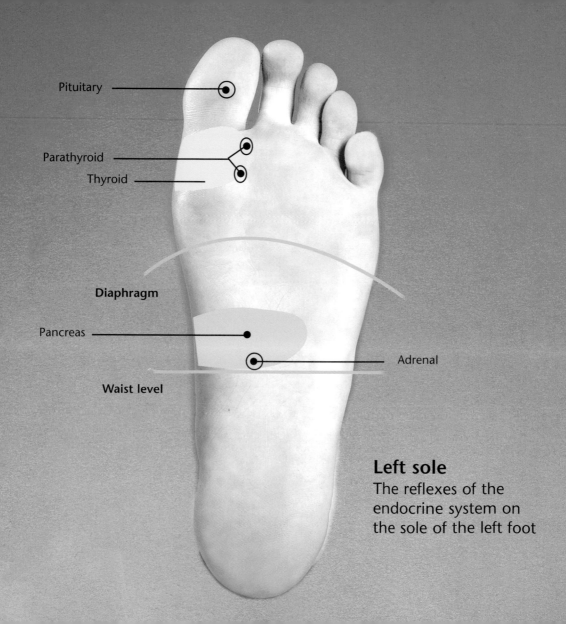

Pituitary

Parathyroid

Thyroid

Diaphragm

Pancreas

Adrenal

Waist level

Left sole
The reflexes of the
endocrine system on
the sole of the left foot

of the thyroid gland is to control the metabolic rate in the body.

The reflex to the thyroid gland is found in both feet in zone one, with the right lobe represented in the right foot and the left lobe represented in the left foot. The thyroid area is over the ball of the big toe and more particularly in the upper part of this area.

The parathyroids are two pairs of small glands embedded in the back of the thyroid gland in the neck. These glands produce a hormone called parathyroid hormone which acts to control the levels of calcium and phosphorus in the blood.

The reflexes to the parathyroid glands are associated with the reflex to the thyroid gland in both feet in the area of the ball of the big toe but on the border of zone one and zone two, i.e. on a level with a line drawn straight down on the sole of the foot from the web between the big toe and second toe. An upper and lower parathyroid reflex will be found in both feet corresponding to the upper and lower glands on both sides of the body.

The adrenals are situated on top of each kidney. Each adrenal gland can be divided into an outer area called the cortex and an inner area called the medulla. The adrenal medulla produces the hormones adrenalin and noradrenalin. The adrenal cortex produces hormones which influence carbohydrate metabolism and the mineral balance in the body, and it also produces additional sex hormones.

Left foot

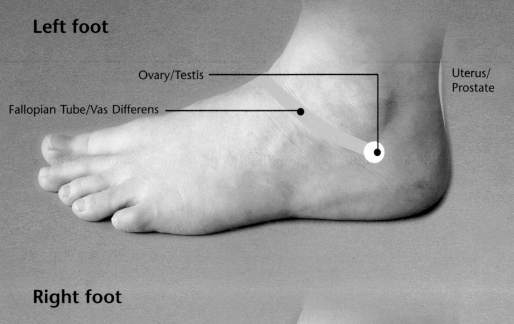

Ovary/Testis

Fallopian Tube/Vas Differens

Uterus/
Prostate

Right foot

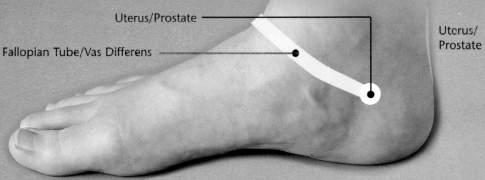

Uterus/Prostate

Fallopian Tube/Vas Differens

Uterus/
Prostate

The reflexes of the reproductive system on the sides of the feet

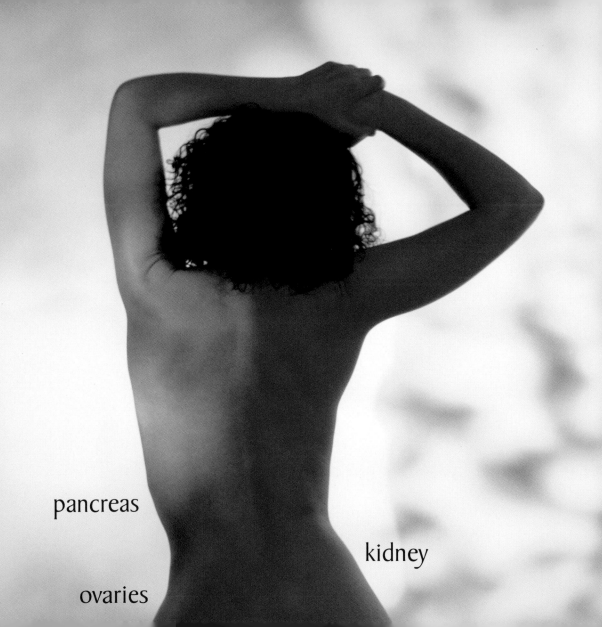

pancreas

kidney

ovaries

The reflexes to the adrenal glands are found just above and slightly to the inner side of the kidney reflexes in zone two of the feet, a little above the waist level of the soles of the feet. The right adrenal gland will be represented in the right foot and the left adrenal gland will be represented in the left foot.

The pancreas is unique in that it is both an endocrine gland and an exocrine gland. The exocrine function is the production of digestive juices which pass down the pancreatic duct into the small intestine. The endocrine function is the production of insulin which acts to lower the blood sugar level. In the body the pancreas is situated behind the stomach just above the waistline.

The reflex to the pancreas is found in both the right and left feet just above the waistline and below the diaphragm in zones one and two on the right foot and zones one, two and three on the left foot. Since in the body the stomach overlaps the pancreas, in the feet the stomach reflex overlaps the reflex to the pancreas on the soles of the feet.

The reproductive glands of the female are the ovaries and of the male are the testes. The ovaries produce the hormones oestrogen and progesterone which control the reproductive cycle and prepare the womb for pregnancy. The testes produce spermatozoa (the male germ cells) and the hormone testosterone which, with the androgens produced by the adrenal cortex, is responsible for the development at puberty of the secondary sex organs and secondary sex characteristics. The two ovaries are situated on either side in the pelvis and are connected via the fallopian tubes to the uterus. The testes are suspended extra-abdominally in the scrotum by the spermatic cords.

The reflexes to the ovaries in the female and testes in the male are similarly placed, being found in an area halfway between the ankle bone and the heel on the outer side of each foot.

The reflexes to the uterus in the female and prostate in the male are placed in an area halfway between the ankle bone and heel on the inner side of each foot.

The reflexes to the fallopian tubes in the female and the vas deferens in the male are found in an area linking the ovary and uterus or testis and prostate gland, respectively, across the top of the foot in front of the ankle bones.

4.   The respiratory system

The respiratory system comprises the nose and mouth, the throat, the larynx, the trachea (the windpipe), the bronchi and the lungs.
The lungs are tree-like in structure with two main branches, the bronchi, dividing into smaller branches called bronchioles before

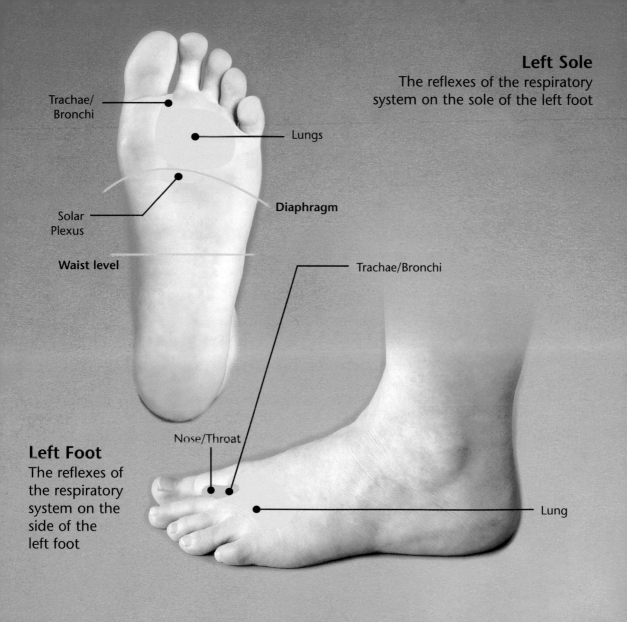

Trachae/Bronchi

Lungs

Solar Plexus

Diaphragm

Waist level

Left Sole
The reflexes of the respiratory system on the sole of the left foot

Trachae/Bronchi

Nose/Throat

Left Foot
The reflexes of the respiratory system on the side of the left foot

Lung

ending in the air sacs called the alveoli. It is within the alveoli that the essential exchange of gases takes place, with the oxygen breathed in being taken up by the blood and the carbon dioxide from the blood being taken up into the air sacs to be breathed out. There are two lungs, one on either side of the thoracic cavity, being enclosed by the ribs and the diaphragm.

The reflex areas to the lungs are found in both feet across all five zones in the area over the metatarsal bones, and both the soles and tops of the feet may show reflex areas.

The bronchi, trachea, larynx, throat, nose and mouth are all air conducting passages and no exchange of gases takes place in these areas.

The reflex area to the trachea is found along the side of the ball of the big toe on both feet, and the reflex area to the bronchus extends across the ball of the big toe from the trachea area into the lung area. These reflexes are present in both feet.

The reflexes to the nose and throat will be found on the top of the big toe in an area just above where the toe joins the foot.

The diaphragm is a dome-shaped sheet of muscle which separates the thorax from the abdomen and encloses the lower surface of the lungs. The mechanism of breathing is a muscular action which involves the movement of the diaphragm.

The reflex area to the diaphragm is found in both feet on the soles, following a line across at the lower level of the ball of the big toe and ball of the foot.

The solar plexus is a network of nerves giving off branches to all parts of the abdominal cavity; it is situated just in front of the diaphragm and behind the stomach. It is sometimes called the 'abdominal brain' since it supplies the abdominal areas as well as the diaphragm and adrenal glands. It is thus a useful area for the relief of tension, stress, fright, anger and nervousness.

The reflex to the solar plexus will be found in an area just below that of the diaphragm on the soles of the feet, in zones two and three on both feet.

5. The heart and circulatory system

A healthy circulation is vital for the good health of all parts of the body and when working on the reflex areas in the feet, the circulation to the corresponding part of the body will be improved.

The heart is a muscular pump which sends the blood around the circulatory system through a series of vessels called arteries, capillaries and veins. The heart is situated centrally in the thorax close to the

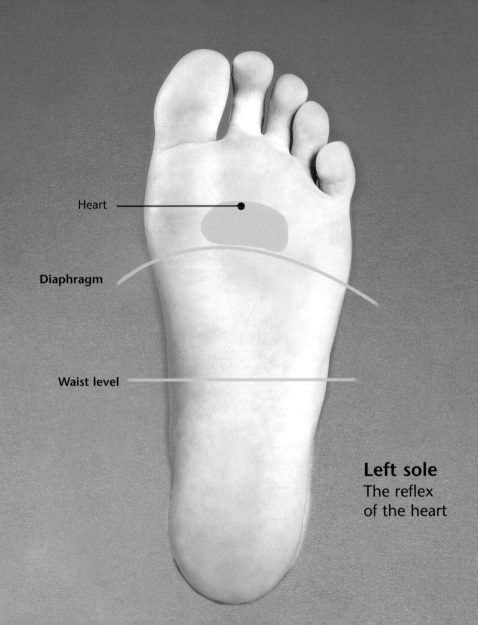

Heart

Diaphragm

Waist level

Left sole
The reflex
of the heart

lungs with two-thirds on the left side of the thorax and one-third on the right side.

The reflex to the heart is a slight exception to the normal determination of reflex areas according to the zone position of the organ in the body. The main reflex area to the heart will be found in the left foot in zones two and three above the level of the diaphragm and overlapping the lower area relating to the left lung reflex on the sole of the foot.

6. The lymphatic system

The lymphatic system is also a circulatory system which works closely with the blood system but is separate from it. Lymphatic vessels are present throughout the body and contain a fluid called lymph, which is similar in composition to blood plasma and contains waste products of cell metabolism which are eventually returned to the blood system. The main function of the lymphatic system is its role as part of the body's defence mechanism.

Lymph nodes are aggregates of lymphatic tissue found in areas along the lymphatic vessels. The lymph nodes are found particularly in the groin, the armpit, the neck, the breast and the abdomen and within

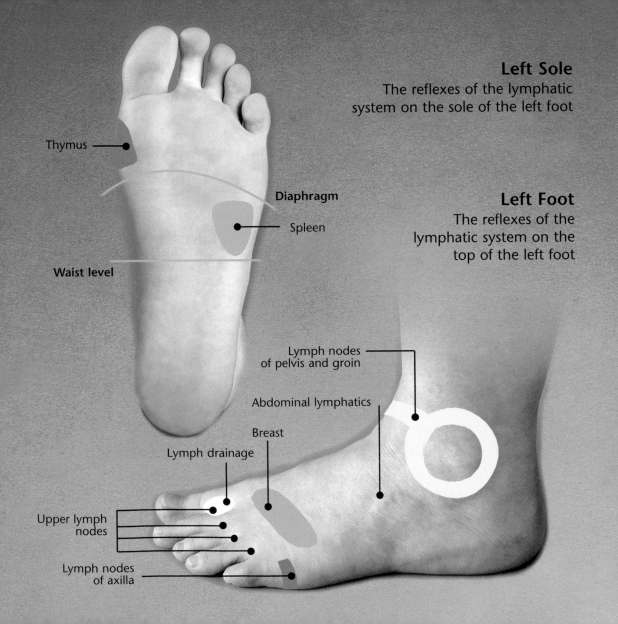

Left Sole
The reflexes of the lymphatic
system on the sole of the left foot

Left Foot
The reflexes of the
lymphatic system on the
top of the left foot

Thymus

Diaphragm

Spleen

Waist level

Lymph nodes
of pelvis and groin

Abdominal lymphatics

Breast

Lymph drainage

Upper lymph
nodes

Lymph nodes
of axilla

these nodes the lymph is filtered and foreign particles and infectious material is ingested by cells called lymphocytes, which help to purify the lymph before it is returned to the blood system via the right and left subclavian veins found in the neck.

The reflexes to the upper lymph nodes are found on the top of the feet at the roots of the toes.

The reflexes to the lymph nodes of the breast are found on the top of the feet in zones two, three and four in the thoracic region lying over the metatarsal bones.

The reflexes to the lymph nodes of the pelvic and groin areas are found on the top of the feet in all five zones in front of the ankle bones and also below and behind the ankle bones.

The reflexes to the lymph nodes of the axilla (armpit) are found on the top of the feet just below the shoulder reflex at the base of the little toe.

The reflex to stimulate the lymph drainage back to the venous system in the area of the neck is found on both feet on the top and sole of the foot at the base of the web between the big toe and second toe. This area can be worked on with a type of pinching action.

The reflex areas between the areas described for specific lymph nodes on the top of the feet will relate to the thoracic and abdominal lymphatics.

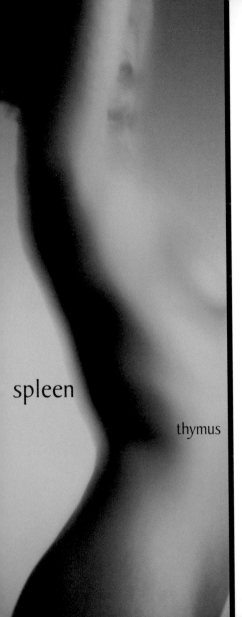

spleen

thymus

The spleen and the thymus are also parts of the lymphatic system. The spleen can act in a similar way to a lymph node by producing lymphocytes, and it is also involved in the breakdown of old red blood cells and can recycle the haemoglobin from these. In the body, the spleen is situated in the left side of the abdomen above the waistline and to the side of the tip of the pancreas. The thymus is important before puberty in helping to develop the body's immune system but its exact function in the adult is undecided. It is found in the body in the thoracic cavity close to the heart.

The reflex to the spleen is found on the sole of the left foot in zones four and five below the diaphragm and above the waistline of the foot.

The reflex to the thymus is found in zone one on both the right and left foot on the sole of the foot in an area over the ball of the big toe.

7. The digestive system

The digestive system is responsible for breaking down the molecules of food ingested into particles that can be absorbed by the blood, which can then be used for the various bodily processes. Any undigested food passes through the digestive system and is expelled. The food ingested passes into the mouth, then down the oesophagus to the stomach, and then to the small intestine and large intestine, with the residue being expelled through the rectum and anus.

The oesophagus leads from the mouth to the stomach and is a muscular tube acting as a passageway to the more important areas where digestion will be carried out.

The reflex to the oesophagus is found on the sole of the foot leading down from below the big toe along the inner edge of the ball of the big toe over the first metatarsal bone to the stomach area.

The stomach is a sac-like structure found in the upper abdomen above waist level on both right and left sides of the body, but with the major part of the stomach more to the left. In this area, food is mixed with digestive juices but no main absorption takes place.

The reflex to the stomach is found on both left and right feet on the soles of the feet above the waistline of the foot and below the diaphragm level. It is found mainly in zones one, two and three in the left foot and zone one on the right foot.

The small intestine receives food from the stomach and the two are separated by the pyloric sphincter, which controls the flow of food between them. It is within the small intestine that the breakdown and absorption of food particles takes place.

The reflex to the small intestine is found in both feet on the sole of the foot below the waistline of the foot and extending down in the area over the tarsal bones in zones one, two, three and four.

The large intestine commences with an area called the caecum and an important valve called the ileo-caecal valve regulates the passage of food from the ileum of the small intestine to the caecum. The large intestine then passes up the right side of the body with the ascending colon which bends round beneath the liver at approximately waist level to become the transverse colon, which continues across to the left side of the abdomen to below the spleen where it becomes the descending colon. This area continues down the left side before turning towards the midline and becoming the sigmoid colon which then leads to the rectum. The rectum is centrally positioned and leads into the anus. The appendix is situated off the lower end of the caecum. The main function of the large intestine is to absorb water and salts to conserve

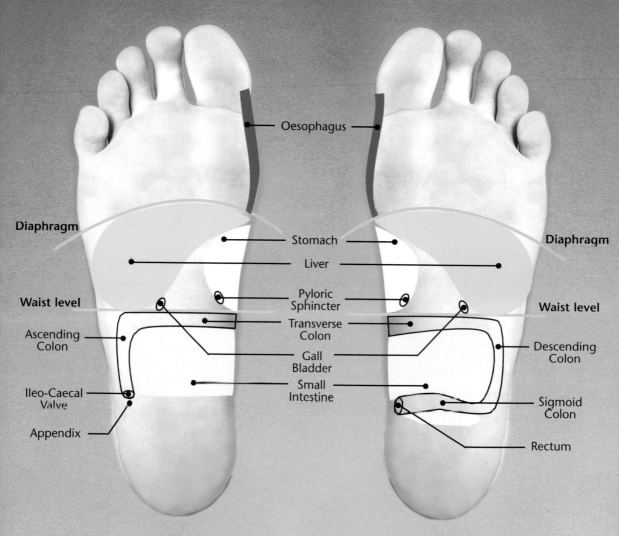

Oesophagus

Diaphragm

Diaphragm

Stomach

Liver

Waist level

Pyloric
Sphincter

Waist level

Ascending
Colon

Transverse
Colon

Descending
Colon

Gall
Bladder

Small
Intestine

Sigmoid
Colon

Ileo-Caecal
Valve

Appendix

Rectum

The reflexes of the digestive system on the sole of the right and left foot the body fluids and it also stores the waste faecal matter until it is expelled.

The reflexes to the regions of the large intestine are found on the soles of both the right and left foot. Commencing on the right foot in zones four and five in the area over the lower tarsal bones with the appendix and ileo-caecal valve reflexes, the ascending colon reflex is found leading up from this area to the waistline of the foot. The transverse colon reflex is found in all ten zones at waist level, with the descending colon reflex found in the left foot similarly placed to the ascending colon reflex in the right foot. The reflex to the sigmoid colon follows an S-shaped path from the end of the descending colon reflex to the inner side of the left foot where the reflex to the rectum is found. A reflex to the rectum may also be found extending from this area up the back of the leg for a short distance on either side of the Achilles tendon.

The liver is the largest organ in the body and amongst its functions are the processes of detoxification, storage of carbohydrates, proteins, fats, vitamins and minerals and the production of bile. In the body, the liver extends across all five zones on the right side and just into zone one on the left side in the area between the diaphragm and the waist. It is tucked in beneath the diaphragm but its lower margin tapers off to give a triangular shape to the liver.

The reflex to the liver is found in the right foot in the area between the diaphragm and the waist. It occupies all five zones just below the level of the diaphragm and then tapers off in its triangular shape to occupy just zones three, four and five above the waist.

The gall bladder is attached to the lower right lobe of the liver and stores the bile produced by the liver. The bile will be released down the bile duct into the duodenum of the small intestine to assist in the absorption of dietary fat and fat-soluble vitamins.

The reflex to the gall bladder is found in the right foot in zone three just below the liver reflex and thus just above the waist level of the sole of the foot.

The pancreas, as discussed in the previous section on the endocrine system, produces various digestive enzymes which pass down the pancreatic duct into the small intestine.

8. The urinary system

The urinary system is made up of a right and left kidney each connected by a ureter tube to the bladder. This is the main excretory system of the body.

The kidneys act as a filtering system which works to maintain the composition and volume of the body fluids. Each kidney is made up of approximately one million microscopic units, called nephrons, which are responsible for the formation of urine. The kidneys are positioned on the posterior abdominal wall at about waist level in zones two and three. The left kidney is situated slightly higher than the right kidney.

The reflexes to the kidneys are found in the soles of the feet at about waist level in zones two and three with the right kidney reflex in the right foot and the left kidney reflex in the left foot.

The ureter tubes are long, thin muscular tubes which convey urine from the kidneys to the bladder.

The reflexes to the ureter tubes are found in the soles of the feet joining the kidney reflex to the bladder reflex and thus passing from zone two across and down to zone one at the inner side of the feet.

The bladder is a hollow muscular organ which acts as a reservoir for the urine. When the bladder is full the desire to pass urine is experienced and the urine is expelled down the urethra. The bladder is situated centrally in the anterior part of the lower abdomen.

The reflex to the bladder is found in both the right and left foot on the inner side of the foot and slightly on the top of the foot. This reflex in zone one is close to that of the lower lumbar region of the spine and is sometimes identified by a slight swelling in this area on the top inner side of the foot.

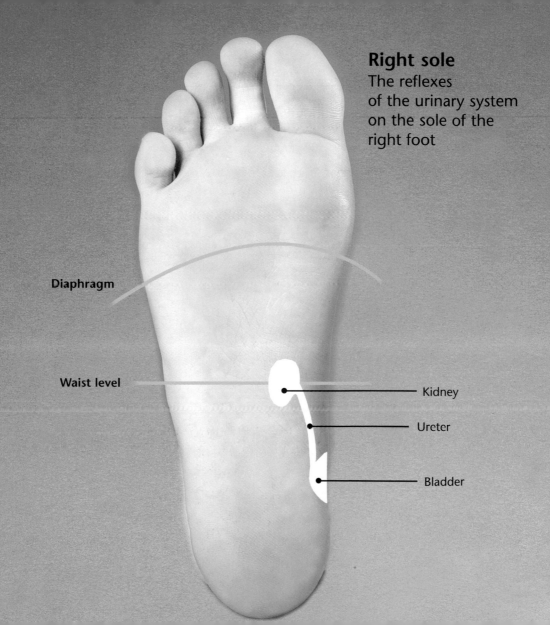

Right sole
The reflexes
of the urinary system
on the sole of the
right foot

Diaphragm

Waist level

Kidney

Ureter

Bladder

9. The skin

The skin is an important excretory system of the body and also acts as a barrier against infection and helps in the control of body temperature. In addition to the many glands present in the skin, many nerve endings are also present allowing the five basic skin (cutaneous) sensations of touch, pressure, pain, warmth and cold.

   The reflexes to the skin are not specifically placed but, since the skin covers the entire body, the different areas of the skin can be reached through the reflexes to the areas underlying the skin.

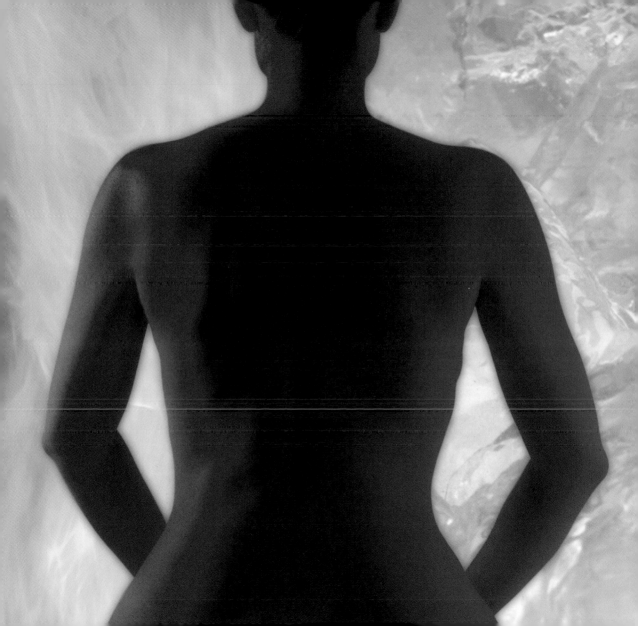

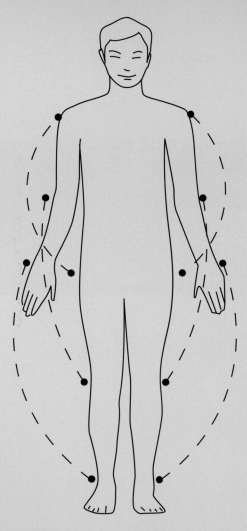

The zones related areas

Zone related areas

In addition to the reflex areas of the feet, a development of the early 'hook work' as mentioned earlier can be applied in connection with the upper and lower limbs.

The arm and leg on both sides of the body can be divided into five zones and zone related areas can be described (these are the same as 'cross reflexes' mentioned by some authorities). These areas link the hip with the shoulder, the knee with the elbow, the ankle with the wrist and also the upper leg with the upper arm, lower leg with lower arm and foot with hand. The relationship exists between the areas on the same side of the body, for instance, right elbow with right knee. The usefulness of these zone related areas is that they may be massaged directly to help a condition when it might be unwise to work directly on the actual area affected. An example of this would be when there was severe inflammation of a joint, such as the knee, when direct massage to the knee might well aggravate the condition, but the elbow on the same side of the body could be massaged directly and might well help reduce the inflammation of the knee. It should be stressed that these zone related areas would be massaged in addition to the massage of the reflex areas in the feet.

What Reflexology is Effective in Treating

By being able to treat all the different parts of the body through the feet, due to the fact that reflex areas to all these different parts exist in the feet, reflexology offers itself as a potential treatment for nearly all disorders. It is important to remember that with reflexology, whatever the condition being treated, all the different reflex areas in the feet will be massaged. However, in certain conditions, certain reflex areas are obviously going to be of greater importance in helping to balance up

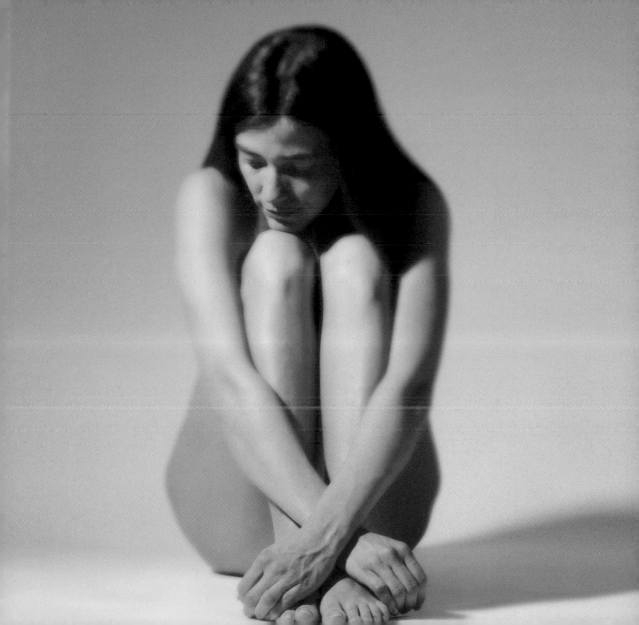

the body and these areas will thus require extra massage.

To help understand the type of conditions which may be treated by reflexology treatment, here are some of the more common conditions seen by practitioners.

1. The head areas: headaches and migraine, stroke (cerebral haemorrhage), Parkinson's disease, multiple sclerosis, sinusitis and catarrh, hay fever, eye disorders (for example, cataracts, conjuncitivitis, glaucoma and so forth), ear disorders (for example, tinnitus and Ménière's disease), toothache.
2. The musculo-skeletal system: spinal (back) problems (for example, slipped disc and pulled muscle), neck problems, shoulder problems, tennis elbow and golfer's elbow, lower back problems, hip problems, sciatica, arthritis and rheumatism, gout.
3. The endocrine system: pituitary disorders, thyroid disorders, adrenal gland disorders, pancreas disorders (for example, diabetes and hypoglycaemia), reproductive gland disorders (female conditions include problems with the menstrual cycle, infertility and the menopause; male conditions include infertility and prostrate problems).
4. The respiratory system: asthma, bronchitis, emphysema.

5. The heart and circulatory system: angina, high blood pressure (hypertension), circulatory problems (for example, chilblains and varicose veins).

6. The lymphatic system: ear infections, throat infections, M.E. (post viral fatigue syndrome), shingles, breast lumps.

7. The digestive system. heartburn, indigestion (dyspepsia), hiatus hernia, ulcers, constipation, flatulence (wind), colitis, haemorrhoids, hepatitis, gall stones, allergies.

8. The urinary system: kidney disorders (for example, nephritis and kidney stones), bladder disorders (for example, cystitis and incontinence).

9. The skin: eczema, psoriasis, dermatitis, acne and miscellaneous rashes.

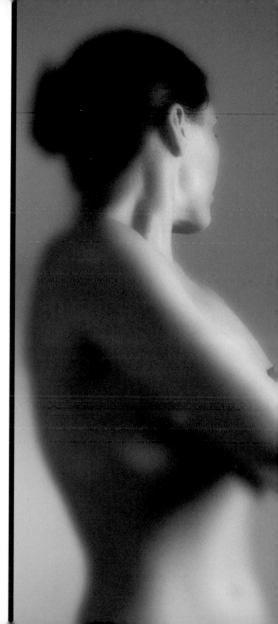

SPECIAL CARE

• Particular care is required with the treatment of diabetes with reflexology due to the possible effect of the alteration of the amount of insulin produced by the pancreas.

• All heart conditions must be treated with extreme care so as not to over-stimulate the heart.

• Extra care must also be taken in treatment of a pregnant woman especially in the first three months of a first pregnancy or where there has been a previous miscarriage.

• Conditions of thrombosis and phlebitis would normally not be treated with reflexology.

There are obviously many more conditions not mentioned above which may well be helped by reflexology. For some of the more serious and complex conditions the trained practitioner may well be able to help in many ways. Cancer has not been mentioned but reflexology can be of benefit in this area. Even if it cannot bring about complete recovery, the overall balancing effect will help to strengthen the whole body up to fight the condition, with the relaxation induced by the treatment helping the patient to cope better both emotionally and physically and also helping with pain relief. In a similar manner, reflexology treatment may be helpful to AIDS patients. With eating disorders such as anorexia and bulimia, the general balancing effect of the treatment and the relaxation achieved may well aid recovery.

Reflexology as preventative therapy

In general, people tend to wait until ill-health develops before seeking help to try and right the disorder, either by conventional means or by one of the complementary therapies. There is now, however, a growing trend towards caring for the whole self more constantly in order to reduce the likelihood of being ill. This caring is not only for the physical body by, for example, eating more sensibly, but also for the mind by, for example, relaxation techniques. Reflexology can be of great benefit as a preventative therapy and offers a means of caring for the whole self. By having treatments at regular intervals, the body can be maintained in a more balanced state with resulting continued good health.

Self-treatment

Although reflexology is best given by a fully trained practitioner to obtain the maximum benefit from the treatment, it is a method which can be used to a certain extent for self-treatment. Many people find the hands more useful for self-treatment than the feet since they are more easily reached.

   Reflexology is harmless, provided that it is applied correctly. To learn how to use reflexology to treat yourself, ask your practitioner to demonstrate the techniques appropriate for your condition. The warnings that must be heeded are not to work too long and not to work too heavily. The tendency with self-treatment is to work on isolated reflex areas related to the condition requiring help but, while this may ease symptoms, the total balancing effect of the treatment will not be achieved.

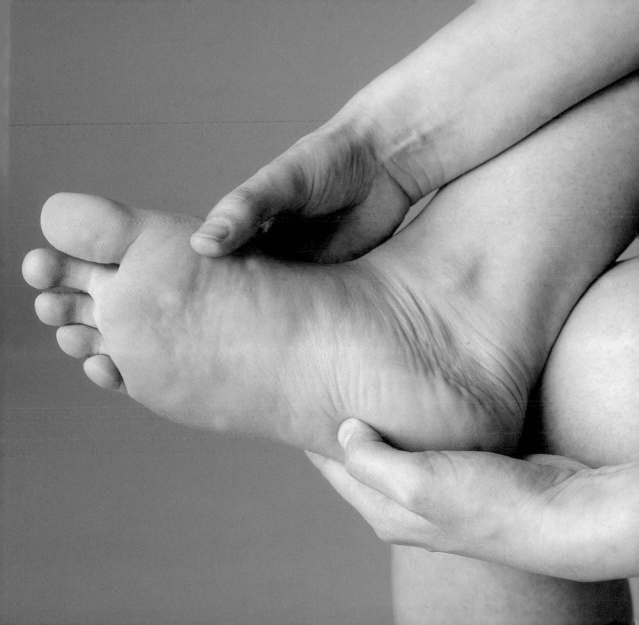

Hand Reflexology

As in the feet, reflex areas are found in the hands corresponding to all the parts of the body and again these are arranged in such a manner as to form a logical pattern of the body in the hands. Most of the reflex points are found in the palms, which can be considered the equivalent of the soles of the feet. The backs of the hands are equivalent to the tops of the feet and the five longitudinal zones described earlier are present in the hands, with each zone corresponding to the area below the digits. The bones of the hands are similarly arranged to the bones of the feet as can be seen by a description of the skeleton of the hand.

The structure of the hand

The bones of the fingers are called phalanges and each finger is composed of three phalanges, except for the thumb which has just two phalanges. The upper part of the hand below the phalanges consists of five metacarpal bones, each extending below one of the phalanges. The remainder of the bones in the hand are called carpal bones and the individual names of the bones are the scaphoid, lunate, triquetrum, pisiform, trapezoid, trapezium, capitate and hamate. The bones are held in place and allowed a range of movements by various muscles, muscle tendons and ligaments.

The reflex areas of the hand

A less detailed description of the reflex areas in the hand will be given than for those reflex areas in the feet since the pattern of distribution of these areas is similar to that found in the feet. Since the hands are smaller than the feet, the reflex areas are found in smaller areas than in the feet and can also be slightly more difficult to detect precisely. However, the principle of the zones still exists in the hands and in whichever zone or zones a part is found in the body, the corresponding reflex area will be found in the same zone or zones of the hands. The transverse zones cannot be so easily applied to the hands since the phalanges and metacarpal bones occupy a substantial part of the hands, with the carpal bones occupying a comparatively smaller area in the hands than the tarsal bones in the feet. Imaginary lines

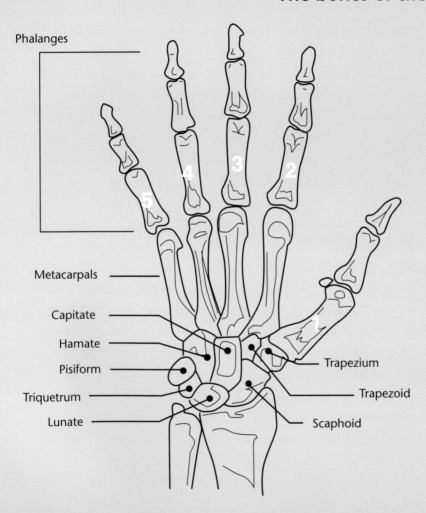

The bones of the hand

Phalanges

4

3

2

5

1

Metacarpals

Capitate

Hamate

Pisiform

Triquetrum

Lunate

Trapezium

Trapezoid

Scaphoid

corresponding to the waistline and diaphragm can be transposed onto the hands to act as a guide to the positioning of various reflexes.

I. The head areas

All the reflexes to the areas of the head are found in regions of the fingers and, as with the big toes, the thumbs correspond to all of the head. The reflex to the pituitary gland is found approximately in the centre of the pad of the thumb and the top of the brain and top of the head reflex area is found at the top of the thumb just behind the nail. The reflex to the side of the brain and side of the head is found down the side of the thumb next to the second finger. The reflex to the face is found on the back of the thumb. The reflexes to the sinuses are found in the second, third, fourth and fifth fingers, both up the palmar surface of the fingers and up the sides. The reflexes to the teeth are found on the backs of the fingers. At the base of the second and third fingers on the palmar side of the hand are found the eye reflexes, with the right eye represented on the right hand and the left eye represented on the left hand. The ear reflexes are found similarly positioned below the fourth and fifth fingers. The reflex to the Eustachian tube is found between the eye and ear reflexes just below the web between the third and fourth fingers and may also be found in a similar position on the back of the hand.

2.   The musculo-skeletal system

The reflex to the spine is found down the inner side of the thumb and hand from the top of the thumb to just above the wrist, with the various regions of the spine again being distinguishable. The reflex to the neck is found around the base of the thumb. The shoulder reflex is found around the base of the fifth finger on the palmar surface, the side of the hand and the back of the hand. Leading down from the shoulder reflex on the back of the hand is the reflex to the arm. The reflexes to the hip and knee are found on the back of the hand on the outer side of the fifth zone close to the base of the fifth metacarpal bone. The reflex to the sacro-iliac joint is found close to the hip reflex but more in zone four on the back of the hand. A reflex to the sciatic nerve is found in all five zones on the palmar surface of the hand close to the wrist.

3.   The endocrine system

The thyroid reflex is found in zone one, below the base of the thumb on the palmar surface of the hand and just below the neck reflex. The

The reflexes of the palms of the hands

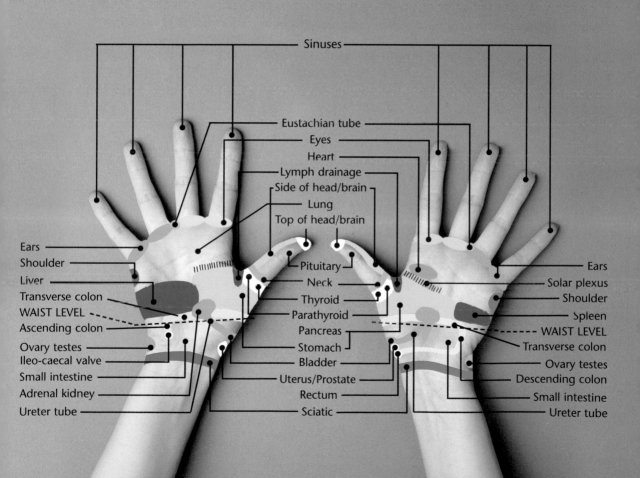

Sinuses

Eustachian tube
Eyes
Heart
Lymph drainage
Side of head/brain
Lung
Top of head/brain

Ears
Shoulder
Liver
Transverse colon
WAIST LEVEL
Ascending colon
Ovary testes
Ileo-caecal valve
Small intestine
Adrenal kidney
Ureter tube

Pituitary
Neck
Thyroid
Parathyroid
Pancreas
Stomach
Bladder
Uterus/Prostate
Rectum
Sciatic

Ears
Solar plexus
Shoulder
Spleen
WAIST LEVEL
Transverse colon
Ovary testes
Descending colon
Small intestine
Ureter tube

The reflexes of the backs of the hands

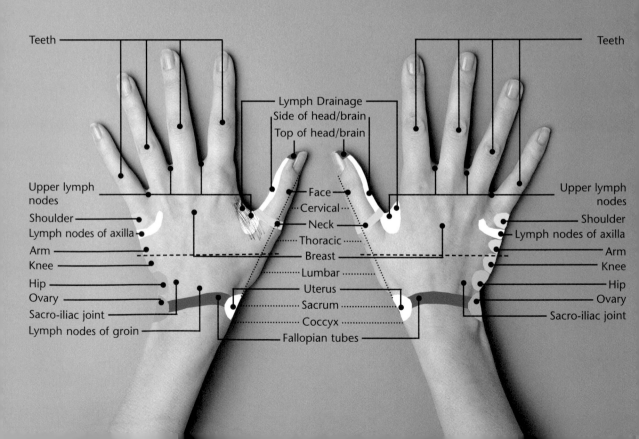

Teeth

Teeth

Lymph Drainage
Side of head/brain
Top of head/brain

Upper lymph
nodes

Upper lymph
nodes

Shoulder
Lymph nodes of axilla
Arm
Knee

Face
Cervical
Neck
Thoracic
Breast
Lumbar
Uterus
Sacrum
Coccyx
Fallopian tubes

Shoulder
Lymph nodes of axilla
Arm
Knee

Hip
Ovary
Sacro-iliac joint
Lymph nodes of groin

Hip
Ovary
Sacro-iliac joint

parathyroid reflexes are found on the side of the thyroid reflex closest to zone two with an upper and lower reflex on both hands. The reflexes to the adrenal glands are found in zone two a little above waist level of the palm of the hand just above the kidney reflexes. The reflex area to the pancreas is found in both left and right hands on the palmar surface in the area between the diaphragm and waist level in zones one, two and three on the left and zones one and two on the right.

The reflexes to the reproductive glands are found on both the palmar surface and back of the hand just above the wrist with the ovary or testis reflex in zone five and the uterus or prostate reflex in zone one. The Fallopian tube reflex joins the ovary and uterus areas across the back of the hand in the female and the vas deferens reflex is represented in this area in the male.

4. The respiratory system

The reflex area to the lungs is found in both hands on the palmar surface below the fingers and in the upper part of the hand above the level of the diaphragm. The solar plexus reflex is found in both hands on the palmar surface at diaphragm level in zones two and three.

5.   The heart and circulatory system

The heart reflex, as in the feet, is found mainly in an area not quite corresponding with the zonal position of the heart in the body but in zones two and three of the palmar surface of the left hand, close to the lung area and above the level of the diaphragm.

6.   The lymphatic system

The reflexes to the lymphatic system are found on the backs of the hands with the reflexes to the upper lymph nodes situated at the roots of the fingers, the breast reflexes situated in zones two, three and four above the diaphagm level and the reflexes to the lymph nodes of pelvis and groin found across all five zones just above the wrist. The reflexes to the lymph nodes of the axilla are found just below the shoulder reflexes on the backs of the hands. The reflex to the spleen is found on the palmar surface of the left hand above the waist level in zones four and five. The reflex area to stimulate lymph drainage to the venous system in the neck is found in the web between the thumb and second finger on both the back and palm of both hands.

7. The digestive system

The stomach reflex is found on the palmar surface of both right and left hands, mainly in zones one, two and three on the left and zone one on the right, above the waist level and below the diaphragm. The oesophagus reflex is in an area joining the stomach reflex from the neck area down the side of the ball of the thumb. The reflex area for the small intestines is found in the palms of both hands in zones one, two, three and four below the waist level and extending down to an area above the wrist. The large intestine is represented similarly in the hands as in the feet, with the ileo-caecal valve reflex on the palmar surface of the right hand in zones four and five a short distance above the wrist, with the ascending colon reflex leading up from this to about waist level and the transverse colon reflex leading from this across all five zones of the right hand and then all five zones of the left hand at waist level. The descending colon reflex leads downwards from the transverse colon reflex in the left hand in zones four and five before turning across towards zone one a short distance above the wrist with the reflex to the sigmoid colon. At the end of this reflex area in zone one is found the reflex to the rectum. As in the feet, the liver reflex is found predominantly in the right hand on the palmar surface in zones three, four and five between the diaphragm and waist level and also in zones one and two in the upper part of this area. The gall bladder reflex is found in zone three of the palmar surface of the right hand just below the liver reflex and just above waist level.

8. The urinary system

The reflex to the bladder is found on both hands on the side and slightly to the back of the hand in zone one, close to the reflex to the lumbar region of the spine. A reflex for the ureter tube leads from the bladder area up to the kidney reflex, which is found on the palmar surface of both hands in zones two and three at approximately waist level.

It is usually found that the reflex areas in the hands are not so sensitive or tender as those areas on the feet. The reflex areas in the hands are useful for the practitioner if for some reason the feet cannot be treated. This might occur, for instance, if there was damage to a part of the foot or infection, in which case the foot would be treated in all the areas possible and the damaged or infected area treated through the corresponding area of the hand.

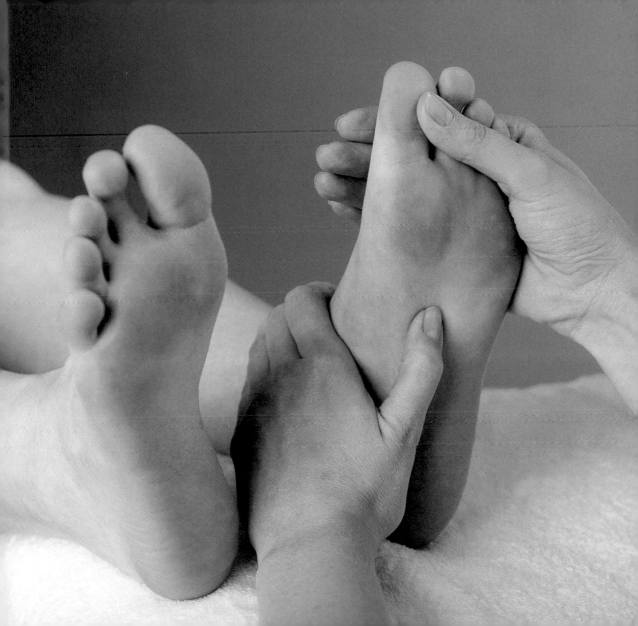

Finding a Reliable Reflexologist

Once the decision to try reflexology treatment has been taken, then the next important step is to try to find a good practitioner of the method.

There are now many training schools for reflexology with a considerable degree of variance between the standards of the courses offered. It is, needless to say, most important that students receive a sound training if they are to see patients on a professional basis.

Most practitioners would agree that the majority of their patients come by personal recommendation. Knowing someone who has been to a particular practitioner and been satisfied is a good way of deciding which practitioner to see. However, if a personal recommendation is not available, then the main training schools are able to give the names and addresses of trained practitioners in the various areas of the country. There are also several representative bodies for reflexology practitioners which provide details of their members – a serious practitioner will be a member of a professional body and will be insured to practise.

Practitioners are allowed to advertise and their details may be found in health magazines, local newspapers and telephone directories. An advertisement does not necessarily mean that the person advertising is qualified, so it is most important that, when contacting someone with a view to receiving treatment, they are asked where they trained, how long they have been in practice and if they are a member of a professional association – anyone properly qualified will not feel embarrassed to give this information.

A final word

In conclusion, it is hoped that, having decided to try reflexology treatment and having found a good practitioner, the results are successful. The treatment does not claim to be able to help everyone and every condition, but the majority of people will benefit. Reflexology must surely be one of the most pleasant treatments available – to lie back for nearly an hour and have all the reflex areas in the feet massaged is a relaxing, health-giving and wonderful experience.

Useful Addresses

UK

The British Reflexology Association

Monks Orchard

Whitbourne

Worcester WR6 5RB

Tel: 01886 821207

Fax: 01886 822017

E-mail: bra@britreflex.co.uk

Web site: www.britreflex.co.uk

The official teaching body of The British Reflexology Association is the Bayly School of Reflexology which can be contacted at the same address. The Bayly School runs training courses at venues in London, regionally, and overseas. Courses are held by representatives of the Bayly School in Australia, France, Kenya, Japan, and Switzerland.

USA

Reflexology Association of America

4012 South Rainbow Boulevard

Box K585

Las Vegas

Nevada 89103-2059

Reflexology Research Project

PO Box 35820

Stn D

Alberquerque

NM 87176